THE INSIDER'S GUIDE TO KETOGENIC DIET AND INTERMITTENT FASTING

Practical Guide on Benefits of Ketogenic and Intermittent Lifestyle to Biohack Your Lean Body, Burn Stubborn Belly Fat, Boost Your Productivity and Energy and how to implement them into your lifestyle

CONTENTS

INTRODUCTION

I want to thank you and congratulate you for downloading the book, "*The Insider's Guide to Ketogenic Diet and Intermittent Fasting: Practical Guide on Benefits of Ketogenic and Intermittent Lifestyle to Biohack Your Lean Body, Burn Stubborn Belly Fat And Boost Your Productivity And Energy*".

This book has actionable information that will help you to tap into the limitless power of the ketogenic diet and intermittent fasting to biohack your lean body, burn stubborn belly fat and boost your productivity and energy.

If statistics are anything to go by, the world is slowly becoming an overweight or obese world with one out of 4 people diagnosed with cancer. But even with the many weight loss programs out there, the number of new cases of obesity seems to be increasing. This probably means there is just something wrong that we are doing that the weight loss programs don't seem to get right. They are just no suited for our body.

Fortunately, all that can be solved with proper understanding of the science of weight gain and weight loss along with the lifestyle that our ancestors were used to for centuries i.e. eating when there was food and going for long hours or even days without food until they could find the next meal. Since the obesity pandemic is a recent phenomenon, this means that there must have been something that our ancestors were doing right with their way of eating even when they really didn't know much about it. This concept is what has been slightly modified for the modern times where food is in plenty and referred to as intermittent fasting.

This is what brings the concept of ketogenic diet blended with intermittent fasting.

A ketogenic diet is a diet that allows you to eat foods that are high in fats, moderate in proteins and low in carbohydrates. I know you are asking; are you not going to get fat when you eat foods high in fat? Well, not really. This combination reduces your carbohydrate intake and replaces it with fat, which puts your body in a constant state of burning fat for the purpose of getting energy, a state referred to as ketosis. On the other hand, intermittent fasting is an eating pattern that consists of periods of eating and fasting that promote weight loss and optimum health. When the two are combined, you get to reduce your general carbohydrates intake drastically while fueling your body with belly fat burning fuel that ultimately helps you to lose weight and keep it off effortlessly as well as attain all manner of other benefits that come with these two.

Is that something you would be interested in? I know you are. If you are tired of trying one fad diet after another because none of them seems to get you to lose weight effortlessly without starving you and keeping it off just as effortlessly, then a blend of these two is worth a try.

This book will show you exactly how to go about it. You will realize that your body is already hardwired for intermittent fasting and staying in a ketosis state i.e. a state where your body runs on fats for energy, which essentially makes weight loss an effortless quest.

Thanks again for downloading this book. I hope you enjoy it!

WE HAVE A SPECIAL FREE BONUS FOR YOU DOWNLOADING THIS BOOK!!!

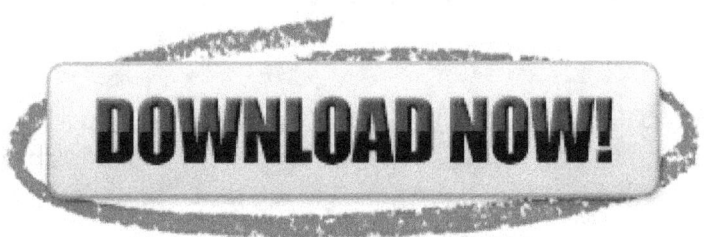

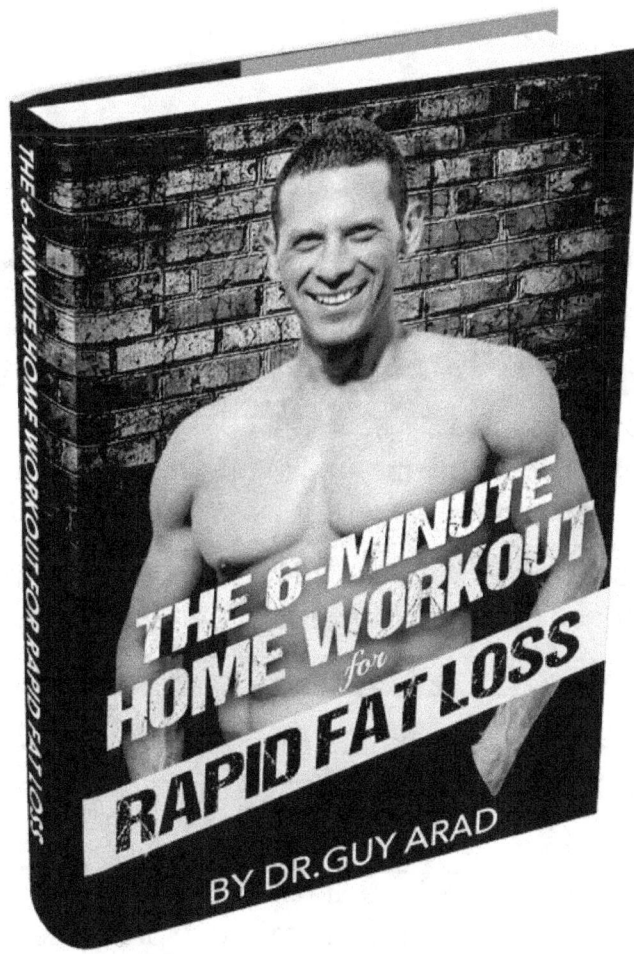

https://suspensionabsolution.com/6-minute-workout-plan

Before we can get to combine ketogenic diet and intermittent fasting, it is important that you understand each one of them in detail.

1. KETOGENIC DIET: A COMPREHENSIVE OVERVIEW

As I have indicated in the introduction, a ketogenic diet is a high fat, moderate protein, low carbohydrate diet that promotes fat burning in your body that can enable you to attain a wide array of benefits, as we will discuss later in the book. Let's start from its very beginning before discussing details of how it works.

HISTORY OF A KETOGENIC DIET

When I first heard about Ketosis last year, immediately all the red lights started flashing in my mind of course as a medical professional.

Most people who heard about ketosis relate it to diabetic ketoacidosis (DKA). DKA is a crisis and happens when a diabetic (Often Type 1) fails to receive adequate insulin.

Therapeutic Ketosis, on the other hand is a very powerful tool to tap into your fat storage, boost energy and productivity and more.

This strategy helped me break my plateau in training and fat loss very fast and why I share it now and also added it to my courses.

The sad truth is most medical professionals are still not familiar with Therapeutic ketosis and the difference between the crisis of DKA and ketosis.

Watch this funny animation explaining ketosis here –click here to watch

Think of the body as a hybrid car that can burn electricity or gasoline for fuel. Our bodies are designed to use two different fuel sources, they can burn sugar (glucose) or fat (ketones).

This is a natural adoption from the Paleolithic Era when humans would cycle through short periods of scattered vegetation and times of a purely carnivorous diet. Summer season would bring spouts of vegetation to our primal ancestors and they would put on some body fat during this abundant time because glucose is a key to fat storage. Winter months would bring little or no vegetation resulting in a diet full of animal fat and meat. This resulted in fat adaptation and required ketosis, burning of fat for fuel.

Our bodies can only store a finite amount of glucose in liver and muscle. Typically this is about 2,000 calories. When you are a sugar burner, you need a constant source of fuel such as glucose that comes from carbs.Any excess sugar will turn into fat..

Our bodies can store large amounts of fat. For example, a 150 pound person with 10% body fat has over 60,000 calories of fat storage!

This is what enabled our ancestors to endure long winters without literally starving to death. Today, we have an endless supply of food all year around...don't we?!?

This means most people never tap into their ketones fuel source and this is the main reason so many of us struggle to lose fat even with diets and workouts...

Studies show our bodies thrive when living off fat (ketones) for fuel. Our muscles will reject glucose in favor of ketones when ketone levels in the blood are high enough. Our brains thrive on ketones and your mental clarity, cognition and memory skyrocket.

Ketosis is defined as a blood ketone level of 0.5 to approximately 6.0. An ideal range is between 1.0 and 3.0. Above a ketone range of about 3.0, you will not see any added benefits.

Dr. Russell Wilder developed the ketogenic diet in 1924 at the Mayo clinic. The purpose of this diet was to treat epilepsy, which it effectively did for some years. But due to the invention of new and improved anti-seizure medications during the 1940s, it fell out of favor (Tracy Putnam and H. Houston Merritt developed the first anti-seizure medication, Phenytoin (Dilantin), in 1938).

In 1994, Jim Abrahams, who was a Hollywood producer, re-publicized this diet when the diet managed to control his son's severe epilepsy. He created the Charlie Foundation, which promoted the diet together with facilitating more research on it. The scientific interest in the diet grew and it was later discovered that it can control and prevent a wide range of diseases as well as help in weight loss.

So how does a diet that was originally meant for fighting epilepsy in children help in losing weight? What's the connection? Let me explain:

HOW DOES A KETOGENIC DIET WORK?

When you are following a ketogenic diet, your carbohydrate intake is limited and this starves your body of its favorite source of energy i.e. glucose. This (the reduced carb intake and subsequent reduction in blood glucose levels) in turn forces your body to get into a metabolic state of ketosis. Ketosis is a natural process that your body initiates when it's low in glucose to burn as energy.

In this state, your body changes its metabolic pathway from burning carbohydrates for energy to burning fat for energy.

So why should the diet be high in fat anyway? Won't fat make you fat? Let me explain this:

THE SCIENCE BEHIND LOSING WEIGHT IN A KETOGENIC DIET

You may be wondering how a ketogenic diet helps you lose weight by encouraging you to consume high amounts of fat. The answer is simple; the popular belief that for you to lose weight you must cut down your intake of fat is a big lie. Eating fat actually helps you lose weight but since I don't expect you to take my word for it, I am going to scientifically explain to you how you can lose weight in a ketogenic diet using the points below:

1. *Eating fat increases your body's ability to burn fat*

    Low fat diets do not condition your body to be efficient in burning fat. They instead create enzymatic machinery that enables your body to efficiently burn carbohydrates. When you take foods high in fats, your fat cells release adipokines hormone, which is a fat-burning hormone that increases the rate at which your body breaks down fat and burns them. So by taking in large amounts of fats, your body is encouraged to burn fat which promotes weight loss. Learn about main hormones involved in your fat burning metabolism here

2. *Consumption of fat displaces the consumption of carbohydrates*

    When you increase your fat intake, your carbohydrate intake automatically goes down because your macronutrient ratio must add up to 100% and proteins are balanced fat when it comes to percentage. So eating more of one macronutrient must automatically lead to a reduction in another.

    When you displace your carbohydrate intake by increasing your fat intake, you set a stage for optimum fat loss. How is that? First, your insulin level lowers because of reduced levels of carbohydrates. This in turn enables your body to easily access fat and burn it as energy, which would have been stored if the insulin levels were high. The new environment encourages fat loss, which increases weight loss and energy in your body.

3. *Fat is filling*

One of the reasons why a high fat diet can greatly help you to lose weight effortlessly is because fat is filling. The reason why many diets are almost impossible to follow is because they leave you feeling hungry, which essentially may make you get tempted to eat. So how does fat make you feel full for it to enable you to reduce the likelihood of snacking or overeating? Well, when the fat you've eaten gets to the small intestines, it triggers a series of signals that include releasing such hormones like CCK and PYY, the two hormones that are very critical in satiety and appetite regulation. This essentially leaves you feeling full and satiated. As a result, you are unlikely to snack between meals or go for a second helping.

4. *The ketogenic diet has a protein sparing effect*

The ketogenic diet advocates for taking moderate amounts of proteins, high amounts of fats and very little carbohydrates. 'Moderate proteins' in this case means that you take just enough proteins to take care of repair and maintenance of muscle mass- not any more. This essentially means that there won't be any excess proteins left after the repair and maintenance of muscle mass. And as a result, you will be assured that the extra proteins won't be converted into glucose/sugar. When this is coupled with the fact that you are taking high amounts of fats and are also burning stored body fat for energy, your body will naturally not need to burn proteins for energy thus the protein sparing effect.

When you pair a high fat diet with low intake of carbohydrates, this ultimately means that the body can metabolize fats due to low levels of insulin as a result of reduced carb levels. That's not all; the fact that the diet entails high fat intake enables the body to start shifting to use of fats for energy, which essentially means that the body can burn both dietary fats and stored fat.

The main aim of a ketogenic diet is to force your body into a metabolic state of ketosis where your body can burn fat for energy. But remember you can't do this through calorie starvation but through carbohydrate starvation. Moreover, keep in mind that fat also has calories; excessive intake of fat will probably make you gain weight as opposed to losing weight. Therefore, this diet of course needs to be accompanied by calorie reduction (you shouldn't expect to consume excess calories from fat and still lose weight!). You will get to learn this as you continue reading.

THE SCIENCE BEHIND A KETOGENIC DIET

For you to understand the science behind a ketogenic diet, you need to first understand some basic biochemistry. Your body generates energy in the form of ATP (adenosine triphosphate) using a process called cellular respiration. This process has three parts namely the electron transport chain, the tricarboxylic acid cycle and glycolysis. Below is a brief description of this process.

The process starts in the cell's cytoplasm where glucose is converted into small amounts of ATP, electron carriers (they are responsible for transferring energy) and pyruvate (which consists of two copies of a three-carbon sugar). The pyruvate molecules then enter into the mitochondrion, which is the cell's energy powerhouse. Here the pyruvate is converted into two-carbon modified sugar called acetyl-CoA and a carbon dioxide molecule. The acetyl-CoA goes into the tricarboxylic acid cycle where a small amount of ATP and electron carriers are generated. In the final stage of cellular respiration, the electron transport chain process occurs where all the electron carriers that were generated from the tricarboxylic acid cycle and glycolysis are combined and used by the mitochondria to produce ATP in a process called chemiosmosis.

Under normal circumstances, human cells start the process of cellular respiration by using glucose that come from carbohydrates in glycolysis. But in a ketogenic diet, the glucose levels are low, which means your body will instead tap into its carbohydrate storage known as glycogen. When your blood sugar levels (glucose and glycogen) are high, you secret lots of insulin to help in transporting the carb into the different body cells. Unfortunately, just as insulin is good, its presence in the body could be just as bad. For instance, when it is in high levels, this essentially means that your body is absorbing as much glucose as possible (include the excess that ends up being stored as glycogen and fat). This essentially means insulin is a fat storage hormone. It doesn't just do that; during the process of initiating glycogen and fat storage, it will inhibit the burning of fat but instead trigger the storage of fat. This is what we want to avoid by making sure that insulin levels are low so that you can ultimately stop inhibiting the burning of fat (which is essentially within the realm of ketogenic diet). You can only do that through limiting the insulin trigger i.e. carb. The good news is that even with glycogen storage, on average; your body will have about 2000 kcals of glycogen, which means this energy will soon be depleted thus prompting your body to seek an alternative source of fuel. When the two energetically accessible carbohydrates are all out, your body will initiate an alternative method to satisfy its energy demand by the name of ketosis. This is only possible because as carb levels decline, the 'fat burning' inhibition brought about by insulin is reduced since there is less insulin being produced in response to carb. This is what you should be aiming at. Let's talk about this in detail:

ENTER KETOSIS: WHAT IS IT ALL ABOUT?

In ketosis, the stored fat is broken down by the liver to release fatty acid molecules and glycerol. The glycerol molecule is usually let free to combine with other glycerol molecules to make glucose in minimal amounts, which add up to the glucose that is used by your brain. The fatty acid molecules are then broken down to ketone bodies more specifically acetoacetate in a process known as ketogenesis. Acetoacetate is normally converted into 2 types of ketone bodies namely:

- *Beta-hydroxybutyrate (BHB)* - Once your muscles become keto adaptive, they convert acetoacetate into BHB, which your brain prefers for fuel since it is water soluble and is thus capable of passing through the blood brain barrier.

- *Acetone-* Acetoacetate can also be converted into acetone, which is mostly expelled as waste and is responsible for the smelly breath that you will get when you start this diet.

The more your body gets into ketosis i.e. a state where it relies heavily on fats as opposed to carbs, the more fats it burns and the greater the rate at which you lose weight. Since ketosis seems to be the secret formula to burning fat, I now you may be wondering how to get into ketosis. Let's discuss how to do that.

HOW TO GET INTO KETOSIS

For you to get into the metabolic state of ketosis, you need to make sure that the majority of your body's energy supply comes from ketone bodies. Your body must break free from the process of glycolysis where your get your energy from blood glucose. When that happens, you reduce your insulin levels greatly thus opening doors for the process of burning fats for energy (which insulin inhibits) and stopping the incessant fat accumulation that's facilitated by insulin.

So the main question here is; how you can get into the state of ketosis? Here are a couple of methods you can use to get into ketosis:

- You can exercise on an empty stomach/fasted workouts. This method helps your body to use up all the glucose in your blood along with its glycogen stores, which automatically results into your body turning to fat as its main source of energy.

- You can restrict your carbohydrate intake to 20 grams or less than that per day. By decreasing your carbohydrate intake, you are cutting the supply of glucose, which is your body's preferred choice of energy. This forces your body to depend on fat as its main source of energy.

✥ Intermittent fasting: This method puts your body in a food starvation mode that cuts down the supply of food, which your body uses for energy. This essentially means that there is a calorie deficit, which your body has to meet by turning to alternative sources of energy. Given that you are essentially taking sufficient proteins to facilitate repair and maintenance of muscles, this means your body won't need to burn proteins (from your muscles) for energy but will instead opt for fat stores thus resulting to fat loss.

So when you try getting into ketosis, how long should you expect to get there?

Well, for starters, a ketogenic diet is not an on and off diet. For you to get into ketosis and benefit from it, you need to be dedicated to it. Normally, you can take anywhere between 2 to 7 days to get into ketosis. But that highly depends on your activity levels, the type of food you're eating and body type. The more active you are, the less time you will use to get into ketosis. Eating whole unprocessed foods that contain less carbohydrate will also help you get into ketosis much faster.

Ultimately, when you get into optimal ketosis i.e. a state where your body becomes an efficient fat burning machine that runs only on fats (ketones) for energy, you should expect lots of benefits some of which we will highlight in the next chapter.

2. BENEFITS OF A KETOGENIC DIET

As I had stated earlier, the ketogenic diet was initially used for controlling epilepsy but that is not all this diet can do. It also helps you to lose weight, increase your energy levels and improve a wide range of health issues in your body. In this chapter, I am going to explain to you some of the benefits that you can expect to see by following a ketogenic diet. Without wasting too much time, let me jump right into it.

1. IT HELPS YOU LOSE WEIGHT AND FAT FAST

The ketogenic diet is one of the most effective methods of losing weight. This is because it uses several methods to tackle weight.

1: First, it puts a stop to fat gain or fat accumulation. Normally, when you eat, your body breaks down the food into their simplest forms, which end up in the bloodstream. These pieces include amino acids, fatty acids and sugars. Immediately these components enter your bloodstream, your body secretes different transport hormones that take them in the cell membranes that need them. Insulin hormone transports sugar and amino acids while lipoproteins transport fatty acids. The two hormones are essential to life. With that being said, insulin is known to store excessive glucose as fat when you consume more carbohydrates than your body requires for energy. The fat accumulation is what eventually causes weight gain and even obesity.

A ketogenic diet puts a stop to this by encouraging a low intake of carbohydrates, which lowers the level of insulin that is responsible for storing excessive glucose as fat.

2: The second method is that it encourages the burning of fat for energy. Here is how. Once your body has decreased its carbohydrate intake, your body lacks its preferred source of energy and it turns to its second best source of energy, which is fat. Remember that the absence of insulin opens doors for fat burning. Therefore, with reduced insulin levels, your body then starts by burning your body fats, which quickly results to weight loss. The good thing about it is that your body will constantly burn fat to meet its daily calorie requirements.

3: It suppresses your appetite and cravings: The other benefit that you can get from a ketogenic diet is the reduction in your appetite. Appetite reduction helps you to avoid over eating. How does a ketogenic suppress your appetite? When you start consuming more fats and fewer carbohydrates, your body stops experiencing blood sugar swings that come from the conventional diet (which is high in carb).

These swings are caused by excess insulin, which is triggered by the intake of carbohydrates. The insulin constantly breaks down all your consumed food, which gives you an appetite to eat more. Since a ketogenic diet has minimal carbohydrates, these swings are reduced and so is your appetite.

A ketogenic diet also suppresses your hunger through the positive impact that ketones have on cholecystokinin (CCK) a hormone that makes you feel full and satisfied.

2. LOWER INFLAMMATION WHICH CAN IMPROVE CHRONIC PAIN, REDUCE HEART DISEASE RISK AND CANCER RISKS

Cancer is one of the deadliest life threatening diseases that we have in the world today. One of the advantages of adopting a ketogenic diet is that it can help you fight and prevent cancer. How does it do this? Let me explain:

Cancer cells normally feed on sugar and as you know, a ketogenic diet limits your carbohydrate intake which means the presence of glucose in your body is minimal if any. Your body cells always function regardless of whether you are using fat or carbohydrates for energy but this doesn't apply to cancer cells. Once your body starts burning fat for energy, they all weaken, decrease in size and possibly die.

The other way a ketogenic diet reduces cancer is by decreasing the production of insulin in your body. Insulin is an anabolic hormone, which helps the cells to grow including your cancerous cells. So when insulin is reduced, the cancerous cells experience a slow-down in growth which slows down even the tumor growth. In short, ketogenic diet is good for controlling cancer and preventing it.

3. IT INCREASES YOUR ENERGY LEVELS

When you adopt a ketogenic diet, your energy levels normally rise. Why is that?

Well, many athletes will tell you that you need to eat carbohydrates if you need to boost your energy levels. To some point, it's true but guess what; fat can provide you with much more energy than carbohydrates can. This is because you cannot store significant amounts of carbohydrates throughout your body but you can do it with fat. Carbohydrates only yield 4 kcal (kilocalorie) of energy while fat yields about 9 kilocalorie of food energy per gram which goes on to show you just how much fat is resourceful when it comes to energy as compared to carbohydrates.

4. IT IMPROVES YOUR CHOLESTEROL

A ketogenic diet is very beneficial when it comes to its impact on your body cholesterol. The diet promotes HDL (High Density Lipoprotein), which is also known as the good cholesterol and decreases LDL (Low Density Lipoprotein) which is known as the bad cholesterol.

Both HDL and LDL carry cholesterol around your blood. LDL carries cholesterol from your liver to the rest of your body and when your LDL level is high, they can form deposits on the walls of the coronary arteries, which may eventually build up and interfere with your blood flow to cause a heart attack or a stroke. HDL carries cholesterol away from the rest of your body to your liver where they are excreted or re-used so if you have lower levels of HDL in your body, the cholesterol in your body may also build up and cause a heart disease.

So how does a ketogenic diet manage to improve the two lipoproteins? It does it by restricting the types of foods that promote the formation of LDL and increases the level of HDL like processed foods and trans-fats. The ketogenic diet does not encourage those kinds of foods, which mean it is easier to control good levels of LDL and HDL in your body.

With all these benefits, I know you want to get started right away. Let me show you how to start following the keto diet shortly.

5. IMPROVED MOODS

6. SHARPER MENTAL CLARITY AND FOCUS

7. SKIN IMPROVEMENTS SUCH AS SOFTER, SUPPLER SKIN OR ELIMINATION OF RASHES/ECZEMA/ACNE.

3. HOW CAN YOU START A KETOGENIC DIET?

Now that you have seen how beneficial a ketogenic diet, the next step for you is to learn how you can start following this amazing diet. Below are a couple of steps you can follow to start following a ketogenic diet:

1. KNOW YOUR MACROS

Macronutrients consist of three nutrients namely carbohydrates, proteins and fats. For you to adapt into a ketogenic diet and be able to enter into the metabolic state of ketosis, you must know how much of each macronutrient you need to consume. The recommended ratio that you should follow is 70% fats, 25% proteins and 5% carbohydrates.

With that being said, the speed at which you will get into ketosis highly depends on your carbohydrate restriction. The more you restrict yourself from carbohydrates, the faster you will be able to enter into ketosis. Anywhere between 20-30 grams of net carbohydrates (total carbohydrates minus total fiber) per day is fine but if you really want to get into ketosis fast, I recommend trying eating less than 15 grams of carbohydrates per day. To calculate the macronutrients in your food, you can use macronutrients calculators from the internet. Below are a couple of links for efficient calculators;

- Download MyFitnessPal app on your phone
- Ruled.me
- Macrofit.com/

2. KNOW THE FOODS TO EAT AND FOODS TO AVOID

One of the difficult parts of changing diets is learning the foods that are accepted and those that are avoided in your new diet, which in your case is a ketogenic diet. Below is an extensive list of foods that you can eat and foods that you can't eat when you are following a ketogenic diet.

Foods to eat

Base most of your meals around these foods:

- **Butter and cream –** eat the grass-fed ones

- **Eggs –** eat pastured or omega 3 eggs

- **Healthy oils** – mainly avocado oil, coconut oil and extra virgin oil, MCT oil.

- **Meat –** turkey, chicken, bacon, sausage, ham, steak and red meat

- **Fatty fish –** mackerel, tuna, trout and salmon

- **Organic ,non GMO Tofu,Temphe ,hemp hearts**

- **Avocados –** try freshly made guacamole or whole avocados

- **Nuts and seeds –** chia seeds, pumpkin seeds, flaxseeds, walnuts and almonds

- **Low-carb veggies –** peppers, onions, tomatoes, radishes, mushrooms, spinach, broccoli and cauliflower.

- **Cheese –** the best cheese are the unprocessed ones which include mozzarella, cream, goat and cheddar.

- **Condiments –** here you are allowed to use some pepper, salt, spices and healthy herbs

Foods to avoid

Basically, all foods that are high in carb should be avoided. Here is a list of other foods to avoid

- **Alcohol-** alcohol can kick you out of ketosis because of its high carbohydrate content.

- **Root vegetables and tubers-** parsnips, carrots, sweet potatoes and potatoes

- **Beans and legumes-** chickpeas, lentils, kidney beans and peas

- **Fruit –** all fruits are good except berries like strawberries.

- **Grains and starches-** cereal, pasta, rice and wheat-based products

- **Sugary foods-** candy, ice cream, cake, smoothies, fruit juice and soda

- **Sugar-free diet foods-** these foods are highly processed and can interrupt your state of ketosis.

3. MAKE A MEAL PLAN

Once you have known what to eat and what not to eat, you need to know how to make a ketogenic meal plan that you will be following throughout the week. A meal plan can be described as a set of meals, which you have planned to prepare on a later date. Below is a three days meal plan that you can follow to get started:

Monday

Breakfast: Ham and cheese omelet and vegetables

Lunch: Shrimp salad with olive oil and avocado

Dinner: meatballs, cheddar cheese and vegetables

Tuesday

Breakfast: A ketogenic milkshake

Lunch: Beef stir-fry cooked using coconut oil with some vegetables

Dinner: Salmon with asparagus that has been cooked in butter

Wednesday

Breakfast: Bacon, eggs and tomatoes

Lunch: Burger with cheese, guacamole and salsa

Dinner: Chicken that is stuffed with pesto and cream cheese alongside vegetables.

This book is about ketogenic diet and intermittent fasting, let's now discuss intermittent fasting before moving on to discuss how to combine the two.

4. TRY THERAPEUTIC KETONES WITH YOUR FIRST MEAL OR BEFORE A WORKOUT.

Therapeutic ketone products are a powder form that contain beta-hydroxybutyrate salts that is easy to mix with water or any other drink (low carb of course...)

If you are practicing intermittent fasting, wait to take ketones until right before your first meal. Here is the Ketones form I take (Use the **code SAS** to get your samples)

5. REDUCE YOUR CARBOHYDRATE INTAKE.

Making a few changes in your carbohydrate intake can have drastic results. Try eliminating sugars in your diet as well as reducing your carbohydrate intake, especially all grains. Grains set off an inflammatory response in your body and intestines and reduce the level of ketones in your body.

6. INCREASE YOUR FAT INTAKE.

Fat is your source of fuel. Eat lots of healthy fats, but look for stable Saturated fats. Avoid omega-6 all together and limit the intake of Poly-unsaturated fats (Trans fats). This means no vegetable oil, Margarine, etc.

Rely on coconut oil, avocado, virgin olive oils, MCTs etc.

7. REDUCE YOUR CALORIC INTAKE AND BEGIN INTERMITTENT FASTING.

Eat all of your food during the day in a 6-9 hour window of time and nothing outside of that timeframe.

8. DRINK MORE WATER.

You need to drink half of your bodyweight in ounces of water per day. The more you drink the better.

9. ADD SALT AND ELECTROLYTES TO YOUR DIET.

Your body releases much of the salt (and associated water) that it holds onto with higher carbohydrate diets so you need to add extra. This means you need to add salt to food, eat high potassium foods like avocado, coriander, parsley, almonds, spinach, Swiss cheese. These all have more potassium per gram than a banana without the added sugar. Supplements are also a good option.

10. EAT THE LAST MEAL OF THE DAY AT LEAST 3 HOURS BEFORE BED AND GET AT LEAST 8 HOURS OF SLEEP.

Eating too close to bedtime interferes with natural human growth hormone production in the body that occurs during sleep. This can stall weight loss.

11. MOVE MORE.

You will experience a surge in energy so use it in your workouts. Our SAS program is a great way to move and practice Total body workouts anywhere in 15 minutes or less.

4. ALL ABOUT INTERMITTENT FASTING

So what exactly is intermittent fasting? Well, intermittent fasting (famously referred to as IF) can be described as a pattern of eating where you are required to eat your food during a specific period and fast for a specific period. Intermittent fasting is different from a diet. This is because it does not tell you which food to eat; it only tells you when you are supposed to eat.

Surprisingly, intermittent fasting is not a new thing. Throughout the evolution, humans have been fasting for two reasons.

- One is lack of food
- And two is because of religious reasons

In ancient times, food was not a guarantee like it is today. This is because your ancestors had no technique for storing food so they ate all they had hunted and gathered hoping that the next day they will get more food. But this didn't always happen. Life was tough. But their bodies had to adapt to such eating patterns i.e. whereby food was not guaranteed to be available at certain times and days. It is only until recently when humans discovered food storage methods so over the years, the body adapted to 'uncertain' and 'unscheduled' eating patterns. To shorten the story, your body is like your ancestors; it is not designed to eat frequently like 3 meals a day. Intermittent fasting is a process that takes you back to how your body evolved to do in the first place.

5. HOW DOES INTERMITTENT FASTING WORK?

For you to have a clearer understanding of how intermittent fasting works, you need to first learn the difference between a fed state and a fasted state.

The fed state is when your body is digesting and absorbing foods that you have just eaten. Basically, the fed state starts when you start eating a meal. Your body spends almost 4-5 hours processing the food and burning whatever it can get from what you have just eaten. During the fed state, it is hard for your body to burn fat since your insulin levels are high because of the readily available food, which your body prefers to use as energy. After the fed state, your body gets to a period where it has nothing to process due to lack of food. This state is known as post-absorptive state. Your body stays in this state up until 8-12 hours after your last meal.

Fasted state comes right after post-absorptive state. In fasted state, your body has no food that it can burn as fuel so it turns to your stored fat as its main source of energy. Before burning fats, it burns much of the glycogen stores after insulin has absorbed much of the blood sugar. If you can fast for long enough to get your body to a point where it has exhausted a large portion of the glycogen stores (this of course happens when your blood glucose levels are low), this can get you into ketosis i.e. a point where your body relies on fats for energy. But since you are not taking dietary fats during this time, you will essentially be burning stored body fat.

This essentially means that if you want to fasten the rate at which you get into the state for burning fats for energy i.e. deplete your blood sugar and glycogen stores; you can exercise to increase your body's energy demands and subsequently burn any carbs very fast. This explains why you can lose fat very fast even when you don't change what you eat but just when you eat.

6. SO HOW CAN YOU FOLLOW THIS EATING PLAN?

Now that you have seen how IF works, it's time for me to explain to you how you can start following this amazing fat lose technique. Intermittent fasting has several different methods, which you can use to implement it. All the methods are efficient and you can choose to go with any of them depending on your preference. Below is an explanation of some ways you can use to do intermittent fasting:

1. DO A 24 HOURS FAST ONCE OR TWICE A WEEK

This is one of the not so hard methods of intermittent fasting. To follow this method, you will need to fast for 24 hours and eat normally for 6 days or 5 days.

A 24 hour fast might seem hard but it is not; the best way to go about it is to start immediately after dinner. For example, if you are through with your dinner after 8 pm, you can avoid eating until the next day at 8pm. That way, you will have done a 24 hour fast.

You can also do the fast from lunch to lunch or from breakfast to breakfast as the results are the same either way. During the fast, you are allowed to take non-caloric beverages like water and coffee but no solid food. As a person who is losing weight, it is extremely important for you to maintain your normal eating habit during your days of feasting. This is because when you over eat, you will be increasing your daily calorie intake, which will obviously inhibit fat loss within the 24 hours.

If fasting for 24 hours is too hard for you, then start with a 14 or 15 hour fast and build your way up.

2. THE 5:2 DIET

This is one of the simplest methods of intermittent fasting. This method requires you to eat normally for five days and then move on to restrict your calorie intake to 500-600 on the remaining two days of the week. During the 2 days of restricted calorie intake, men should take 600 calories and women 500 calories.

The other good thing about this method is that the 5 days do not have to consecutively follow each other. You can choose to restrict your calorie intake on Tuesday and on Friday. In short, you are allowed to choose the days you wish to restrict your calorie intake.

3. THE 16/8 METHOD (LEAN GAINS PROTOCOL)

If you prefer to fast and feast every single day, then this is your method. Basically, this method requires you to fast for 16 hours in a day and feast for the rest of the day which is 8 hours. This is one of the natural ways of implementing intermittent fasting. You can try to fit in at least 2 or 3 meals in the 8 hour period of feasting.

The best way to execute this diet is by not eating anything after you've had your dinner and then skipping breakfast. For instance, if you finish your dinner at 8 pm, you should eat the next day at 12 noon after skipping breakfast. You will have completed a 16 hour period of fasting and the best part is that most of that time you spent while sleeping. During the fasting period, you are allowed to take non caloric beverages like water and coffee.

4. THE WARRIOR DIET

This was popularized by Ori Hofmekler who was a fitness expert. In this eating plan, you are supposed to fast for 20 hours and eat within a 4 hour period. The best way to go about this is to fast all day and eat a huge meal at night. What you eat is also very critical to this method as its philosophy is based only eating natural foods.

This method allows you to under-eat when you are fasting so you can take small amounts of raw fruits, fresh juice and vegetables. During the 4 hours feasting phase, you are allowed to take one large meal that consists of natural foods, which are whole and unprocessed.

5. ALTERNATE-DAY FASTING

This is one of the easiest and realistic methods of intermittent fasting. This method requires you to have an up day and a down day, which means eating very little on one day and eating normal on the next day. On the down day, you need to limit your calorie intake to one fifth of your normal calorie count per day. For instance, if as a woman you take 2000 calories and as a man you take 2500 calories, on your down day you should take 400 and 500 calories respectively.

This method is perfect for your weight loss ambitions, as it can lose you about two and a half pounds of weight per week. But this is if you cut your calories intake by 20 to 35 percent.

All the above methods can make you lose weight so long as you discipline yourself to eat fewer calories and not to overeat during your eating periods.

7. HOW DOES INTERMITTENT FASTING AFFECT YOUR CELLS AND HORMONES?

When you start practicing intermittent fasting, a couple of things happen to different parts of your body. For instance, your cells initiate important repair processes and at the same time, they change your genes expression. On the other hand, your hormone levels change in order to make your stored body fats more reachable. Below is a summary of what occurs in your body during fasting:

- Insulin: when fasting, your levels of insulin will actually drop dramatically because of lack of carbohydrate intake. The reduced secretion of insulin makes your stored fat much more accessible.

- Human Growth Hormone: During the intermittent fasting process, the growth hormone normally increases which is a good thing for fat loss and muscle gain.

- Cellular repair: when you are in a fasted phase, your cells initiate some cellular repair processes. One of the processes is autophagy where the cells digest and get rid of old and dysfunctional proteins, which normally build up inside the cells.

The above changes are responsible for various health benefits of intermittent fasting.

8. INTERMITTENT FASTING AND WEIGHT LOSS

Intermittent fasting is a powerful weight loss tool. That's one of the reasons why its popularity has grown over the years. So how does intermittent fasting help you lose weight?

It starts by first cutting out the weight gain channel, which is eating excessive calories that end up being stored as fat in your body. It does this by promoting the consumption of fewer calories, which enables your body to get the amount of food it needs to use as energy without necessarily having a surplus to store as fat.

So unless you compensate your lack of eating during fasting with excessive eating, you will generally be taking fewer calories and according to a 2014 review study, this can lead to major weight loss. In this review, the researchers found out that intermittent fasting reduces body weight to about 3 to 8% and this is over a period of 3 to 24 weeks.

The same review also examined the rate of weight loss and found out that people doing intermittent fasting lost 0.55 pounds or 0.25kiligrams per week and this rate increased to 1.65 pounds or 0.75 kilograms when they were doing alternate-day fasting. They further discovered that by doing intermittent fasting, you can lose 4 to 7% of your waist circumference which indicates that you will lose belly fat when you are following intermittent fasting. These results show just how effective intermittent fasting is when it comes to weight loss.

But as you have seen above, there are also other factors that influence weight reduction in intermittent fasting. These factors include changes in hormone levels that facilitate weight loss, lower insulin levels that reduce fat storage and the increased release of fat burning hormone called norepinephrine or noradrenaline. With that being said the main reason why intermittent fasting is one of the best tools for weight loss is because it helps you consume fewer calories.

When you follow this way of eating, you can be sure to derive a number of benefits such as those we will discuss in the next chapter.

9. BENEFITS OF INTERMITTENT FASTING

Fat loss in intermittent fasting is great but the benefits of it go way beyond just weight loss. Numerous studies about intermittent fasting have been done on both animals and humans and they have shown that this method does not just have weight loss benefits but also metabolic health benefits that can lead to a longer and a healthier life. Below are a couple of benefits, which you can get from this method:

1. DECREASES INFLAMMATION

One of the risk factors for inflammation and cardiovascular diseases is homocysteine. Homocysteine normally reacts with biologically essential molecules in your body especially proteins. When it reacts with proteins, it causes damage specifically to the folding of your important proteins like structural proteins, growth factors, receptors, immune proteins and enzymes. It then leaves them with a less optimally functional configuration. This causes oxidative damage, which results into inflammation in the endothelium among other parts.

Intermittent fasting helps decrease inflammation by decreasing the levels of homocysteine in your body. How? Homocysteine is a midway substance in the metabolic pathway that is between methionine and cysteine (which are amino acids). Vitamin B12 and folate are important when it comes to the transition of methionine to cysteine. If you have a deficiency of either vitamin B12 or folate in your body, the aforementioned transition results into an increase in the level of homocysteine, which leads to inflammation. Intermittent fasting increases the level of folate and vitamin B12, which decreases homocysteine and eventually inflammation. And that's how intermittent fasting helps reduce inflammation.

2. IT LOWERS YOUR RISK OF TYPE 2 DIABETES

Type 2 diabetes has been an illness that has been growing over the years. Its main risk factor is high blood sugar levels, which causes insulin resistance. This means that type 2 diabetes can be controlled by anything that can lower blood sugar levels and insulin resistance. One method that does that effectively is intermittent fasting.

Intermittent fasting has major benefits for insulin resistance and usually leads to a reduction in your blood sugar levels. Intermittent fasting is all about limiting meal frequency and limiting the intake of calories.

The combination of those two keep your blood sugar in check, which controls the amount of insulin produced in your body and improves insulin resistance. In simple terms, lack of frequent supply of food reduces the need for the production of insulin to transport glucose to the cells.

In one human study on intermittent fasting, the blood sugar was seen to reduce by 3 to 6% and the insulin was reduced to 20 to 31% which is an impressive reduction. Check the human study here:

So as you can see intermittent fasting can help you control type 2diabetes and prevent it from occurring if you don't have it.

3. IT MAKES HEALTHY EATING SIMPLE FOR YOU

Sticking to a healthy way of eating is very hard. It requires you to plan a head, come up with a healthy meal plan and then later execute it by cooking for yourself. That is a lot of work and that's why it is hard for people to maintain a healthy lifestyle.

One of the benefits of intermittent fasting is how it makes healthy eating easy. It does this by reducing the frequency of your meal times as most of the times you are required to eat 1 or 2 meals a day as compared to the regular 3 or 6 small meals. This reduces the work of planning ahead, cooking and even cleaning up after your meals.

4. IT CAN EXTEND YOUR LIFESPAN AND HELP YOU LIVE LONGER

How much and how frequent you eat has much more influence in your body than just losing weight. When you are practicing intermittent fasting, your body reacts by making changes in your cellular that help you prolong your lifespan.

Firstly, fasting changes your body's source of energy from glucose to fat. Glucose is a dirty source of energy and this is because it produces way more reactive oxygen species than fat; plus burning glucose for energy encourages fat storage which causes obesity that leads to diseases. On the other hand, burning fat for energy helps you avoid varies diseases and automatically extends your lifespan.

Intermittent fasting also helps you to regenerate your immune system, which also increases your lifespan. It does this by a process known as autophagy in your mitochondria. This process makes your body start to eat itself in order to clean out the damaged parts and that's how intermittent fasting helps you to live longer.

5. CELLULAR REPAIR

When fasted, your cells initiate cellular repair processes. This includes autophagy, where cells digest and remove old and dysfunctional proteins that build up inside cells and we will have more stem cells that repair damage.

6. GENE EXPRESSION

There are changes in the function of genes related to longevity and protection against disease. Genes that are responsible for anti-inflammatory effect will be turned on and others that cause negative effects will be turned off.

10. HOW CAN YOU LOSE WEIGHT FASTER IN INTERMITTENT FASTING?

When it comes to losing weight in intermittent fasting, some people find it easy and others find it challenging. But you shouldn't be worried as there are a couple of methods which you can use to lose weight faster in intermittent fasting. Check them out below:

☞ First, for you to lose weight fast, you must practice to eat only when you're hungry and eat until you are satisfied. When you overeat or eat unnecessarily, you not only slow down your weight loss process but you also hinder the effectiveness of intermittent fasting. This is because your excessive calorie intake will replace all the fat lost during the fast.

☞ Secondly, you should move more if you want to lose weight fast in intermittent fasting. Here are some great ideas of how to do that:

(i)   Take the stairs to your office instead of getting on a lift

(ii)   Alight from a bus one stage before your home stage and walk home

(iii)   Walk to the store

(iv)   Do some walking in the morning

☞ Thirdly, you need to exercise if you want to lose weight fast. Fasting reduces your insulin levels, which facilitates the natural burning of fat for energy. So when you add exercising into the equation, the energy demand goes up which translates to more fat being burned. The best time to exercise is when you're almost ending your fast or before taking your first meal after fasting.

Now that you have a good understanding of ketogenic diet and IF, I know you understand that both can help you to reduce your calorie intake, carb intake and ultimately reduce your insulin levels, which in turn opens doors for fat burning i.e. ketosis. So how can you blend these two diets to derive the most benefits? We will learn that next.

11. HOW TO INCORPORATE INTERMITTENT FASTING AND A KETOGENIC DIET

The ultimate way of losing weight is by combining intermittent fasting and a ketogenic diet. This combination can easily double your weight loss and help you reach your ultimate goal of leading an energetic life, lose belly fat and gain a lean body faster. How exactly can they do that?

When you adopt intermittent fasting and you are on a ketogenic diet, you derive many benefits in regards to weight loss and increased energy. One of the reasons why this happens is because of how the two processes support stable sugar levels. Let me break it down to you.

One of the reasons why people gain weight is because of eating excessive calories that end up building up in your body as fat. Your blood sugar levels play a huge part in this because the higher they are, the more your extra sugar is stored as fat and the higher your appetite is since all the food has been absorbed.

Intermittent fasting starves your body from getting food, which lowers your insulin levels, due to lack of incoming food. When this happens, your body is given a chance to burn fat and the good thing about it is that your appetite decreases since there are no blood sugar fluctuations. When doing intermittent fasting only, your insulin will rise up again during your eating period since your food choice is not limited. But when you combine it with a ketogenic diet, your eating periods will also promote fat burning for energy (because ketogenic diet is low in carb, which subsequently results to low insulin secretion and subsequent fat burning), which will give you that double effect on weight loss.

In short, when you combine the two methods, your body will constantly be in the metabolic state of ketosis meaning you will be losing weight all day and all night. Exercising can also increase your weight loss but be careful not to bite more than you can chew

12. TOOLS AND ACTIONABLE STEPS FOR YOUR USE

Download this PDF with practical and simple strategies you can start right away without doing any more research, calculate your macros, calories for weight and fat loss

Try therapeutic ketones to help you with smooth and quick transition into ketogenic lifestyle and ketosis

Let me tell you right now that some of the ideas and tips you will discover here will sound controversial and maybe shocking at first or different from we were all taught over the years.

I work and being coached by some of the most paradigm breaking people who developed these 'bleeding edge' concepts after years of research and trial with lots of people around the world. I can tell you that most of the conventional ideas and guidelines didn't work for me and take lots of time and cause frustration for many (eat before your workout ,get your protein immediately post workout with carbs etc. ..) and that's mainly why most people quit on their fitness and health programs .

The worst diet on the planet killing people is...Low Information Diet!!

You probably heard it before and deep inside you already know that you have to educate yourself, invest some time in yourself and your body, and learn about your foods and nutrients.

 Download fitness pal app for free and see what's the breakdown of your foods and meals in calories, protein, fat, fiber, carbs etc. .

Yes, it takes some time to adjust and change but remember this: Every big and life changing Change is messy at first, uncomfortable in the middle and gorgeous at the end. Do it! Otherwise where are you going to live?!?! ?

Before we go and calculate the amount of calories tailored for your body during Phase I and phase II let me talk here about couple of key principles and benefits of Intermittent Fasting (IF).

Intermittent fasting (IF) is currently one of the world's most popular health and fitness trends. People are using it to lose weight, improve health and simplify their healthy lifestyle and longevity.

Many studies show that it can have powerful effects on your body and brain, and may even help you live longer and avoid common diseases like diabetes, blood pressure, cancers and more.

Before we show you how to calculate your daily calories and Macros for your IF let's review couple of important principles:

#1. You will need to have a negative energy/calories balance if you want to lose weight or lose fat. Meaning you will have to work out at least 3-4 times a week and decrease your calorie intake in order to get real results. The reason most people who are eating healthy foods and still not losing weight is too many calories and especially carbs that spike the insulin levels and blunting fat burn .

#2. If you really want to go after the body you desire you will have to cut on sodas, juices, dairy and wheat (yes, even wholegrain breads etc. ...) and go low on Carbs. Most of them cause weight gain, inflammation and bloaty belly look, hormonal imbalance (decline in Testosterone and increase in Estrogen) among other issues. We will show you how to cycle through low carb days and high carb days so you change your metabolism and become a fat burner machine!

#3. You will have to incorporate more veggies especially green leafy veggies like broccoli, spinach, kale etc. . . Ideally 70-80% plant based or more will help you lose weight & fat better and get leaner. You will also improve your recovery from workout sand aches and pain if you give it a shot. You will also poop more and get rid of the toxins.

#4. If you want to switch your metabolism and become a FAT Burner beast for life here is what you should do: Intermittent fasting coupled with low carb /high fat/ high protein diet - go and do your workout fasted. Why? Because this will change your metabolism into fat burn rather than burn food that you ate pre workout. Yes ,you can drink your coffee (add some coconut oil and cinnamon to it ,drink water with lemon as you wake up but don't eat .

 Post workout try and push your meal for about 1 hour or even till noon time so your body keeps burning fat (not muscle). Eat mostly protein, fat and very small amount of carbs. Wait till next meal till you are very hungry.

It will take you about 21 days but once you do it, you become a fat burner for life, no carb/sugar cravings anymore and you enjoy from a bunch of other health benefit (regulate blood glucose, cancer prevention and more).

Rely on health fats like avocado ,coconut ,olive oil sources for fat and stay away from carbs even quinoa, oats etc. during the next 4 weeks .

These ideas will help you keep your insulin and cortisol levels low and avoid weight and fat gain.

 # 5. Drink at least half of your bodyweight (Lbs.) in ounces of water per day. For example if you weigh 150 lbs. you should drink a minimum of 75 ounces or about 2Liters a day but consuming about 1 gallon a day will help you faster with weight or fat loss .Drink your water away from food not to dilute stomach acids and interfere with optimal digestion and absorption of nutrients . Add 12 ounces of water for every 30 minutes of workout and 12 ounces of water for every caffeinated drink. Shoot for 1L in the morning and then 2 L during the day.

A great way to do that is start with s big Green smoothie you sip over an hour or so.

#6. I love fruit too …but if you want to lose fat and weight and lean out you will have to cut back and maybe eat them post workout. If you do eat them just don't drink them in your smoothies …so at least you get the fiber from the fruit. A lot of people throw so many fruits in their morning smoothie and just spike their insulin sky high and can't understand why they can't lose weight.

#7. Meal planning and prepping – invest in local produce; go organic as much as you can. Plan your meals, maybe once a week and prep your food. Make it simple, the fewer items you have on your plate the less calories you eat {period}. Use glass containers instead of plastics, especially for hot food. Carry healthy snacks with you always so you don't give in for bad treats and unhealthy snacks.

#8. Cheat once a week – yep, I said it! The quickest way to give up on your new lifestyle and nutrition habits is to deprive you of certain foods for too long.

One meal will not affect your results as long as you are sticking with your plan the rest of the week. Psychologically this will even boost your results and workout the next day, don't feel guilty about it. Be happy and enjoy it! Remember you earned it by doing the hard work during the week!

#9. Gratitude – when you look at your food, take a minute, slow down, don't watch TV or YouTube or check your social media … can you be grateful for the food on your plate? Let's make every meal spiritual and thank the universe/god for that food on your plate in front of you. You will know and feel if you should eat it.

HOW TO CALCULATE YOUR BASAL METABOLIC RATE (BMR) AND KNOW YOUR CALORIES INTAKE FOR YOUR BODY AND GOAL?

It's easy and really simple! Let's get started

#1. HOW TO CALCULATE YOUR BASAL METABOLIC RATE (BMR)

Go to http://www.myfitnesspal.com/tools/bmr-calculator and enter your height, weight, age and sex for free.

Now you will need to download the **my fitness pal** app (FREE) on your phone.

It looks like this in your app store

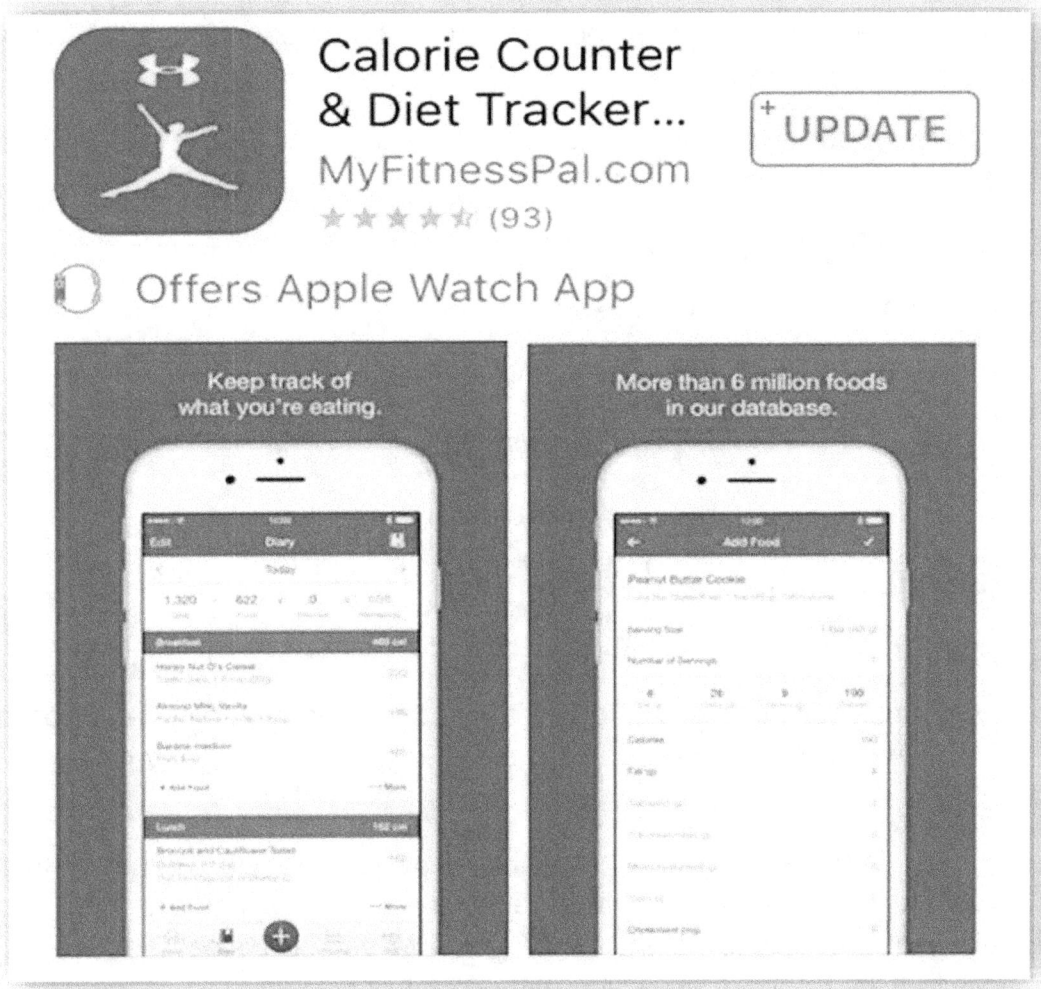

Let's see how it works

Say you are a 45 years old male, 6 feet tall and weigh 200 pounds

Your estimated BMR is: 1,830 calories/day.

Another example is a 40 years old woman, 5 feet weights 140 pound

Your estimated BMR is: 1,227 calories/day

#2. FIND YOUR MACROS' PERCENTAGES AND DAILY INTAKE IN GRAMS.

The most effective way to lose body fat, have more energy and longevity is Intermittent Fasting (IF) with low carb intake /ketogenic.

Meaning you will rely on healthy fats like avocado, olive oil, coconut oil, healthy lean protein sources and fiber.

Inside fitness pal you will go to Goals=> Calorie and Macronutrient Goals and then enter the calories and adjust your carbs, protein and fat so your daily carb intake is below 100gr /day and making sure you get to 100% by adjusting your fat% and protein % accordingly.

So in the above mentioned example Say of a 45 years old male, 6 feet tall and weigh 200 pounds

Your estimated BMR is: 1,830 calories/day.

A reasonable choice is   15% carbs =69gr

                            30% Protein=137gr

                            55% Fat=112gr per day.

#3. YOUR EATING SCHEDULE FOR INTERMITTENT FASTING

Fasting For 16 Hours Each Day

This simply means you will finish eating at say 9.00pm each evening, and not eat again until lunch (around 1.00pm) the following day. So all you are really doing is missing breakfast.

The next 8 hours are your eating window. During this time you can have either 2 or 3 meals, depending on your need for calories and nutrients. If you are fairly sedentary, 2 meals will probably be sufficient. But if you are very physically active, or are an athlete, bodybuilder or sportsman, you will probably need 3.

This method is excellent for anyone who wishes to gain solid muscular body weight whilst staying lean (or even reducing body fat). But of course in this instance it's vital that most of your meals are composed of high quality, nutrient dense foods, with plenty of protein, complex carbs, good fats, and lots of vegetables. You will still take your supplements in the morning and drink tons of water (Try and alkalinize your water using lemon, etc.)

#4. CARBS CYCLING, AVOIDING METABOLIC ADAPTION AND CHEAT NIGHTS..

Carb cycling helps your metabolism and body adjust to burn calories and body fat.

So you want to aim for 3 out of 4 days to go for IF and on the fourth day eat some carbs ideally not from grains initially, so sweet potato, yams are great.

Psychologically it's really important to give yourself one night a week to cheat and eat whatever you like..!! Awesome. Right?! You will be back to your routine and will have easier time to adjust to your new health routine and lifestyle.

Remember we can't outrun or outperform our fork..!!

Here are some cool links and resources about intermittent fasting and turning into a fat burning lean machine (and avoid cancer etc. ...)

Dr.Mercola: Benefits of IF

http://www.youtube.com/watch?v=xyNTTY2zyrw&list=FLCeGpnVouBa6c5cu5ytTgJg&sns=em

Mark Sisson: http://lewishowes.com/podcast/mark-sisson/

Intermittent fasting for lean body transformation

https://www.youtube.com/watch?v=6QOJpQTl640

ABOUT THE AUTHOR

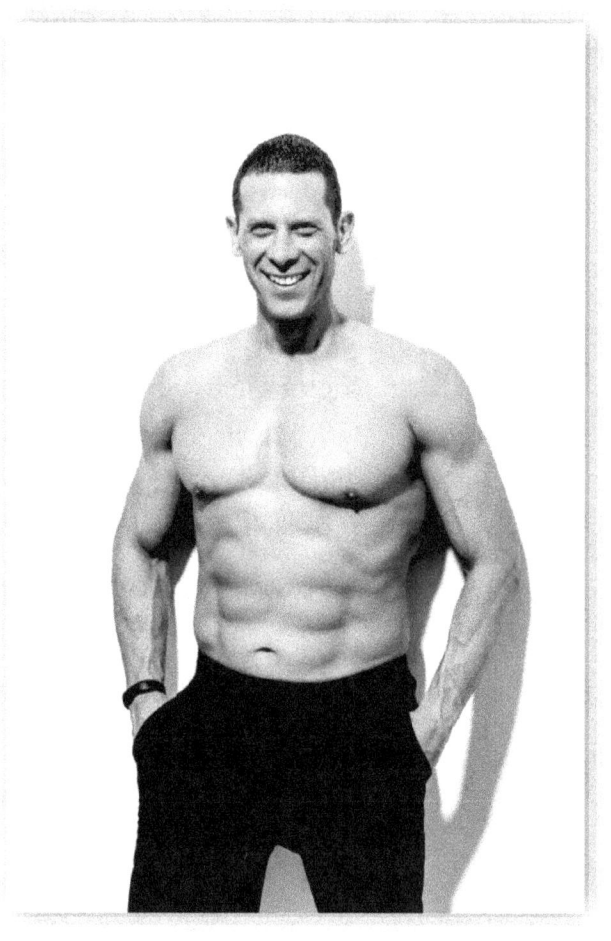

Guy Arad is an ex-Israeli military, dad, entrepreneur, Vet surgeon and functional Suspension Coach and expert; (yes, this is me after a kick ass session)

I especially love helping busy people get results from their workouts and save lots of time using suspension workouts and also helping parents spend more time with their families using our online platform around whole foods, intermittent fasting and ketogenic lifestyle.

I am super passionate about helping people hacking their health using plant based whole foods, intermittent fasting and ketogenic lifestyle as well as coaching on Suspension workouts and kettle bells using HIIT .

I live in Vancouver BC, Canada with my wife, 2 girls, Mila (our puppy), 2 cats, 1 guinea pig and recently a baby bearded dragon.

I would love to hear your story and please feel free to text me (778-558-0322) or hit me on voxer (guyaradster) regarding our nutrition program and recommendations and all fitness questions as well.

You can get my FREE report and 6-minute workout plan and lots of other goodies here just go to➔

suspensionabsolution.com/6-minute-workout-plan

Train hard, live pure!

Guy

CONNECT WITH ME ON THE SOCIAL NETWORKS :

Follow me on snapchat : https://www.snapchat.com/add/guyaradster

Follow me on Instagram: https://www.instagram.com/guyaradster/

Follow me on Facebook: https://www.facebook.com/mysuspensionbody

Grab my free report for Ketogenic diet and 3 wicked Core workouts here

http://suspensionabsolution.com/6-minute-workout-plan

CONCLUSION

Thank you again for downloading this book!

I hope this book was able to help you to understand how to unleash the full power of ketogenic diet and intermittent fasting and maybe give it a try ..!!

Now is your turn to use the information in this book to take action.

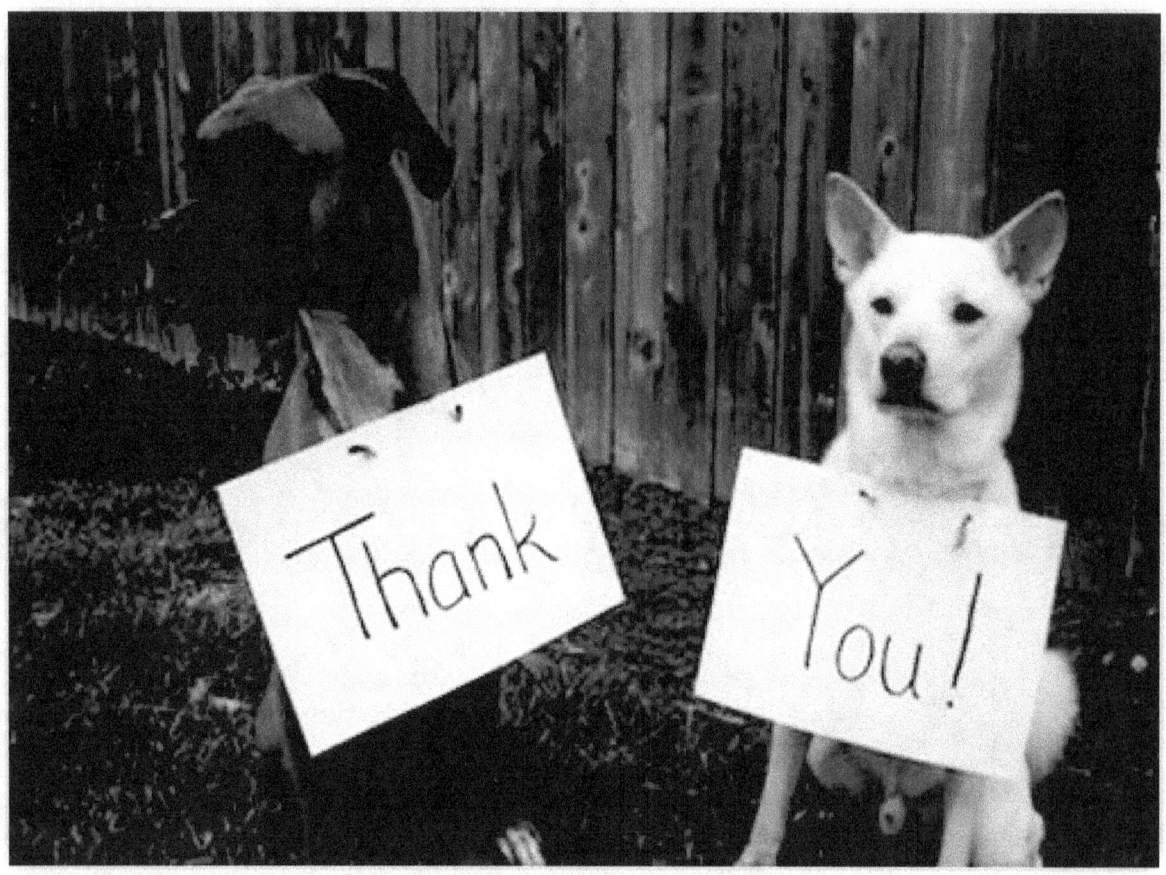

Finally, if you enjoyed this book, would you be kind enough to leave a review for this book on Amazon?

Click here to leave a review for this book on Amazon!

Thank you and good luck!

Guy Arad